F I N A L E
F I T W I T H F I N A L E

The last diet & lifestyle book you'll ever need

By Finale Fitness

DISCLAIMER:

This book is intended for the original purchaser only.
Any duplication, replication, distribution, or sales
not directly from http://www.fitwithfinale.com or our
authorized partners are against our terms and subject
to legal action. This book is for informational
purposes only and isn't intended to diagnose, treat, or
prevent disease nor is it a substitution for
professional medical advice of any sort. Any and all
claims in this book are not guaranteed and are made
based on individual results and author opinions. All
results vary. You must be 18 or older to follow this
book. Any and all activities and ideas you participate
in from, or inspired by this book are at your own sole
discretion and leave you, and only you, fully liable
for your own actions and the outcomes that occur.

Contents

Introduction

We would like to welcome you. You are here because you want to live a more prosperous, successful, and healthier life. You are here because you want to take control of everything around you and be the best **YOU** that you can possibly become. Changing your diet and ultimately changing your entire life can feel like the most daunting task you have ever been put up to. But, it is the most important thing to do in your life if you strive to have outstanding quality and longevity.

Food is something that we will have to live with for the rest of our lives. You cannot live without eating, so it is essential to make sure you understand everything about it. Just think, if we can't live without food and it's so imperative to human life, why would we choose to eat horrible things that can turn our bodies into perfect environments for awful diseases to flourish? We have created the many deadly health problems that face the human race just from dieting choices alone. Here at Finale we give you simple, accurate, and on-the-spot solutions about what you need to eat, why you should eat it, and how you can change yourself forever.

Your diet is more than just changing the amount of fat or muscle you have on your body. It's more than just looking good in the mirror. Your diet controls your entire well-being. Your diet is a reflection of your mental toughness, patience, and will. Having a good (or bad) diet affects your health, relationships, career, outlook on life, prosperity, and your perception of things around you. A better diet is the most important change you can make in your life that will make you healthier, happier, more alive, and much more vibrant for the future.

And who could ever ignore the effects a great diet has on the way you look? Let's be honest, by being thin and having a low body fat percentage, you are perceived as more attractive. Six-pack abs, lean faces, ripped muscles, and sexy bodies are the most desired body features in the world.

Here at Finale we understand this, which is why we constantly remind you that by following our lifestyle, you will develop physical traits you have never had or haven't had in a long time. You'll start to see your jawline again and your six-pack will be on its way back more and more each day. Whether you'd like to look better, feel better, do better, or be better, you'll quickly realize you'll accomplish everything by following Finale.

Again, we'd like to welcome you to the last book on diet and lifestyle you will ever need. **Enjoy!**

Mindset is Everything

When you set forth to accomplish any goal, it is at least 80% mental. Whether you plan to get a promotion at work, save for a vacation, buy a new car, purchase a new house, or budget for those new pair of cool sneakers, your mind goes through changes and processes that must come together to help you accomplish these goals. Without a superior mindset, your goals to lose weight will be absolutely miserable.

Think about that person who is always negative. The person you know who looks at the bad in **EVERYTHING**. Are they happy? Of course not. Are they fun to be around? No. Do bad things happen to them? YES! Our lives are nothing but a complex bundle of events that are perceived by us as good, bad, helpful, horrible, opportune, or detrimental. Look at it like this: for every 200 people that receive a past-due bill and cry, moan, and sulk in their own pities, there will be that one special person who looks at the same bill and gets inspired, motivated, and determined to be greater than their current situation.

Those are the Bill Gates' of the world. Those are the successful entrepreneurs we see on TV. Those are the fat to flab stories we read about. Those are the obese people turned fitness models. They get driven to never have to look at a past-due bill again, or another roll on their stomach. That's why less than 1% of people in the world are rich, famous, and/or immensely successful. When's the last time you met someone insanely rich or insanely ripped? They're rare, but they have finally figured it out, their **mindset is everything**.

Now we're sure you're thinking, how does all of this correlate with **ME** and my diet? Well, it correlates very well. How many times have you succumbed to the temptations of bad eating? Have you ever eaten something only to regret it and feel sluggish and miserable afterwards?

Of course you have! How many times have you felt depressed, down, or uninspired by your body or life's events and turned on the "I don't care" switch? So then you say, "Whatever," or make up an excuse and eat all the cookies, cakes, sodas, high calorie meals, and anything else you can get your depressed hands on. Take it from us, this is **THE WORST** thing you could possibly do. This is like digging yourself in a deep hole while simultaneously covering your head with dirt. By allowing yourself to eat unhealthy while you already feel depressed, stressed, or down, you are setting yourself up for an unhealthy, disastrous pattern. When you **ALREADY** feel bad about yourself, you eating crap will only reinforce these negative feelings and make your mindset much, much worse.

An unhealthy lifestyle is a vicious cycle with a few distinct, but related phases:

1. You eat like crap

2. You feel like crap

3. You start to look like crap

4. You feel and look the worse you have in a while

5. Your self-esteem drops

6. You get so down you become depressed

7. Your goals become non-existent

Because of all of this, you keep picking up weight, your quality of sleep becomes horrible, and 2 years later you're 100lbs heavier, more depressed than ever, and your face, eyes, body, and health have aged tenfold.

You have to change your anger and depression into a vengeance for success and not an opportunity for your sorrows and downfalls. Just because you're depressed doesn't mean the world will stop. People go to work, achieve their goals, and become fitter, leaner, happier, sexier, and richer while you are sitting in your room dwelling on a few things that have happened in your life. It's important to realize that depression is a stagnant, lonely place you have to lift yourself out of.

Sometimes it may feel that life is raining on you, nothing is going right, everyone seems mean, and your overhead seems impossible. What you have to realize is that you probably aren't as bad as you think. Start by counting your blessings and realize you have the power to change your life and your outlook **RIGHT NOW.** You don't have to be another overweight, depressed, diabetic, ugly, and miserable person. You have to dig deep within yourself and find that inner fight, that person you know you can become in every aspect of your life.

The Two P's

Positivity and Progression

As we just discussed, positivity plays a major role in achieving your success in dieting and looking great. Many people look at cravings, hunger, or dietary setbacks as a bad thing. The real job in all of this is to stay positive. Realize that having cravings are completely natural. After all, you've probably eaten anything and everything at one point in your life, sort of getting your mind and body used to junk foods and no structured eating plans. There was one point where you acted on these cravings and you actually went out and got the ice cream.

Now you will fight these sensations and realize that looking and feeling amazing feels much better than a fattening snack that lasts 5 - 10 minutes. Junk food has **NO LONG-TERM BENEFITS. NONE.** A candy bar is only as good as it lasts and that's not a long time. Look at the big picture and you will have no other choice but to eat healthy!

Progression is important in all aspects of life. Whether you are trying to get a report done for school or work, or you need to finish the business plan for your new business, you must progress every single day. Progressing on your diet is learning that **YOU CAN** beat cravings daily, knowing **YOU CAN** eat healthy, knowing **YOU CAN** stay positive; that's the type of progression you need. Trucking through obstacles, low points, mental roadblocks, and financial burdens gives you that progressive mindset that everything is possible, everything is always transcending, nothing is stable, and life is liquid.

Life Conditioning

As a society we have conditioned ourselves to promote food with happiness and celebration. Birthday parties, nights on the town, promotions, banquets, and almost every source of celebration calls for food. Food needs to be looked at as a source of fuel, because at its core that **IS ALL IT IS**. Your body **doesn't care** how good or bad broccoli, chicken, candy bars, or cookies taste. It just wants nutrients, fuel, and energy!

This life and societal conditioning has given everyone a sense of entitlement when it comes to great tasting foods. We're sure you've heard the many excuses against healthy eating such as "vegetables are nasty," "fruit really isn't my thing," or our favorite "I'm a meat and potatoes guy." Well, your body doesn't care if you don't like broccoli because your body **LOVES** broccoli. It doesn't care if you don't like oranges, it **ADORES** oranges. Your body doesn't care if you like candy, it **HATES** candy.

Your body would yell at you if it could for every time you eat loads of fatty meats and fries without any vegetables and fruits. Or the times when you go the entire day without eating, and when you finally do, it's a hot dog, chips, and a soda – your body would scream. Eventually, your body finds a way to yell and scream at you, by developing nasty illnesses like diabetes, heart disease, and cancer.

Why on earth have we lost sight of our discipline with diet? Chances are **you do things you don't want to do every day**. You work, do chores around the house, run errands, take care of kids and loved ones, and take time out of your day to please other people. Basically, you sacrifice every single day to better suit your life and/or the others around you. So why would you look at your diet any differently?

Yes, we know you would rather snack on a candy bar than a banana, but why would you do that to your body? We're sure you'd rather stay home and not go to work, but you still show up for your work obligations. We're sure you'd rather take the money you pay for your car payment and use it for shopping, yet you pay your car note. We're sure you don't feel like running errands, grocery shopping, and doing laundry — but you do it! So why would a **HUGE OBLIGATION** like your diet be any different!?

Looking at it this way, you **ALREADY** have what it takes to be thin, slim, and trim. Think about it - you have discipline! You go to work every single day, you may have spent years and years in school, you have stayed late at work, you've missed fun nights on the town to head into work early, or you've given up lunch with friends to run errands. You possess the discipline, the work ethic, and the focused attitude it takes to be a great dieter.

What is really harder? The 4 relentless years it took to get your degree, the decades you have/will devote to your career, the sacrifices, loss of sleep, and stress of raising children, the overtime you do for extra money or more recognition at work, or choosing a banana over a candy bar for snack? Come on, don't make dieting seem impossible — life is much, much harder! You have what it takes, you do harder things every single day!

Actually, dieting is more important than all of these things because you can't live well and prosperous if you are sick. You can't be who you want to become or stay who you are if you feel ugly, overweight, unhealthy, and stressed out. It's much harder and sometimes impossible to run errands and do laundry if you are constantly out of breath, plagued by stomach aches, or even worse: diagnosed with heart disease, stroke, or diabetes.

Make dieting just as important as your job or source of income and we bet you will see a much better you! It's all about conditioning yourself back into realizing that **a good diet is an obligation.** Just like making money, taking care of your kids, and paying taxes, you **must do it.**

Maybe you're already immensely rich or successful. You didn't get like that from being lazy. Maybe you are an amazing parent who busts their tail at a job you dislike to raise your beautiful children. **DO YOU REALIZE HOW MUCH SACRIFICE ALL OF THIS TAKES**!?

Next time you want to eat a piece of cake or a big cheesesteak, just think, "I can become so financially successful, devote my life to raising kids, or sacrifice my time and mental energy for school, work, and errands but I can't grab a piece of fruit instead of cake?" When you put it in perspective, dieting is easy!

You Can Change

As hard as it may seem, or as hard as life beats you down, there is **ALWAYS ONE THING YOU CAN CHANGE** and that is **YOUR OUTLOOK**. You may not be able to shed those 135lbs **RIGHT NOW** or buy a million-dollar home **NEXT WEEK**, but **RIGHT NOW** you can change **YOUR OUTLOOK**. Changing your outlook on your life, your

current situation, and the events that have
led up to your current situation do not cost
money, isn't restricted by some outer being,
and is **COMPLETELY IN YOUR CONTROL.**

Of course, you could look in the mirror
and say, "I'm fat, ugly, and I need to lose
100lbs. I'll never do this and I hate that I
look like this," or you can look in the mirror
and say, "Wow, I got myself here, but life
isn't over. I'll lose all of my extra weight,
reclaim my life, and reward myself by going to
the beach, strengthening my romantic/personal
relationships, and moving toward my career
goals as a newer, healthier me." Do you see
the switch? If you had to bet, which type of
person would you pick to achieve their goals
in weight loss?

All we are in life are the decisions,
changes, and habits we make throughout all the

days, months, and years of life. The reason someone is obese (barring any illness) is because they decided to eat a lot, not exercise much, and continue to do that over a long period of time. The opposite is also true — the reason a fitness model looks the way they do is because they chose to eat healthy, exercise more, and devote themselves to becoming fit over a long period of time.

When you talk to someone successful in any area of life, it is because they made consistent decisions and changes in their life to better suit them for success in what they were after.

You have to be honest with yourself. Why did you gain weight? What brought you here? You'll find out it was your habits, lifestyle, and mindset. Maybe in college you partied too much, ate out a lot, and didn't care about nutrition. Maybe throughout your career you put your career first and forgot to take care of yourself and your body. It could also be your responsibilities of family, or hardships in life like divorce and death, that put you in a mental state where you made bad decisions about eating and exercising. Whatever it was, you need to be honest with yourself about why you got there. Once you are, the door to success is opened.

From now on, there is **ABSOLUTELY NOTHING** that should stop you from keeping your positive mindset. There **will be** times where you feel like life is beating you down or that something isn't going your way. In no way shape or form does that mean to give up. Embracing hardship allows you to realize the past, analyze the present, and make better for the future. Being down can be a good thing —

it will teach you how to stay up when you're successful.

All in all, going through some difficult times makes you a more appreciative individual when you finally do achieve what you are after. Gaining weight, filing bankruptcy, getting a divorce, losing your job, having a health scare, or losing a friend to an argument doesn't mean you stop living your life! You aren't dead! Life goes on every second, minute, hour, and day after you go through these things, and you must **STAY POSITIVE**!

You are Special, Too

One of the chief complaints we hear from people is that they aren't like these other successful people who achieve their goals. Yes, Bill Gates is special, Oprah Winfrey is special, your favorite fitness model is special, but so are you! They are ordinary people just like you who have decided that they wanted to **CHANGE** and make their lives richer, happier, and more purposeful.

Every single one of us was born with a brain that gives us common sense. Common sense is **ALL YOU NEED** to be successful with your goals. Sure, going to Harvard, being a genius, being a corporate heir/heiress, and having awesome genetics may make life much easier, but most of the successful people in the world haven't boasted such credentials. Common people live extraordinary lives every single day because they have decided to live with control, efficiency, and dedication to their goals.

As you should know, **EVERYONE** has the same 24 hours in the day. You think you're too busy

to cook a few healthy meals? Busy
entrepreneurs, serial inventors, and Fortune
500 executives have the same amount of time as
you: except they have to run some of the
largest and most innovative corporations and
companies on the globe. Think you're too busy
or going through too much hardship? There were
reports that Oprah Winfrey was born into
poverty, was molested by multiple family
members, and still became one of the most
influential media figures in human history.

You see? There really isn't a need to
complain. You are a special individual with
your own array of talents, strengths,
weaknesses, and characteristics. You truly
have what it takes to be successful — you're
unique! You're not too busy or going through
too much; many people are doing much more with
their 24 hours than you. So get out there, get

what you want, lose weight, and achieve your goals!

A Reason for Change

Your body is an amazing machine. Think about it, your heart beats 40 million times a year, your lungs never stop giving you quality air, and your liver, kidneys, and digestive system never take a break. Your body works for you 24/7.

With something so loyal to you, why would you do it harm? If you're 40 years old, that means your heart has performed over 1.6 billion beats! Why would you continue to damage it with horrible foods, bad habits, and no exercise? You are literally betraying the one thing that is built to keep you alive and well!

Always remember, junk food serves no long-term benefit. Sure, a candy bar is good then and there, but once it's gone so is the satisfaction. You're just left with a load of sugar and calories, a bigger gut, and a worse mindset.

Whenever you eat something, be honest with yourself. Ask yourself, "What will this do for my body?" By asking yourself this question, you can be constantly reminded that your decisions on food now, will affect you in the near future. Don't allow yourself to fall off the bandwagon.

One of the most fascinating points ever made about the importance of health is the accountability it takes to face health problems. If you put yourself in a situation where you have heart disease from a horrid lifestyle, lung cancer from long-term smoking, or a limb amputation from diabetes, you are faced with that problem every single day. You can't run from health problems; you take your body with you everywhere you go!

Most problems aren't like that. If you hate your job, you can quit or get a new one. If you don't want to see your ex again, you can move to another city. Or if you want to escape the pressures of bills and life, you can sell all of your belongings and move to some tropical location! But if you are diagnosed with heart disease, you have to live with that day in and day out, wherever you are and whatever time of day it is. You can't run to another city to get away from that problem; it will always stick with you. Your diabetes in America will be the same diabetes in China.

You can't sleep it away and you can't take a vacation and let it clear out. You will have to face the fact that you have damaged your body forever. You get one body — after that, it's gone. That is why, for the love of your body, future, sanity, and longevity, you must change . . **TODAY**!

Getting Started with Finale

There are many ways to achieve weight loss. But not every way is efficient, effective, and safe. Here at Finale, we focus on education which helps you to understand why and what you do for your body. In this book you will find everything you need to lose your weight, look incredible, and be as healthy as you can possibly be.

We stand by and promise you that this will be the last diet book you will ever need. Barring any extreme and unlikely advancements in science, there is no one food, or one **SPECIFIC** diet that will **MAKE** you live longer. All it takes is a balanced lifestyle of healthy eating, exercising, and positive thinking. The way we approach things is simple: you will have 10 rules to follow at all times of your life. Follow these 10 rules and you will be set for weight loss, great health, and longevity. We also give you more knowledge about fitness, cheat meals, diet myths, and extra rules to better educate you on what it takes to be lean, fit, healthy, and sexy. One thing is certain; don't pay attention to the magazines that come out every single month with "something new." People are already living to their hundreds and it's not because they followed some magazine, fad diet, or avoided gluten, carbs, chicken, or beef. It's because they lived an overall healthy lifestyle like the one we are about to show you.

Food Labels

The greatest thing about the modern food industry is the intense regulation it is put under. In the United States and many other modern nations, it is the law for food manufacturers to provide a nutrition facts table on most packaging of food items. This is **IMPERATIVE** to the success of your healthy lifestyle. **YOU MUST KNOW WHAT YOU ARE EATING.** That way you can't complain and avoid mistakes to what you are putting in your body. No one would jump in a pool of ice and complain it's cold. So why someone would look at a horrible food label, consistently eat that kind of food, and then complain they are fat makes no sense. It's all about accountability.

Food Scale

The only thing we strongly suggest you buy that you may not already have is a food scale. You can buy one from virtually any grocery/super store. This will allow you to measure the amount of food you are eating.

Don't worry; you don't **need** a scale most of the time, but it will become very helpful when you are measuring out things like meats or following serving sizes of foods that aren't clear. But again, with the nutrition facts and serving sizes on the food labels, a food scale isn't an absolute necessity.

10 Rules for Life

These are Finale Fitness' 10 Rules for Life. This is the core of the program and will need to be followed adamantly so you can make the changes necessary to follow our diet and lifestyle.

1. Calorie Rule

BMR + Activity Level + Goals = Result

Calories, calories, calories. You hear about them constantly. There is a good reason you do; calories are **THE MOST ESSENTIAL** part of **ANY** diet. **ANY** good diet that makes you lose weight **HAS TO BE** lower in calories. That's right, for all of you no carb, no meat, gluten-free, sugar-free people – the reason you see any weight loss on your diet is because you're simply cutting out an entire food group, which cuts calories! There is nothing magical about any of these types of restrictive, fad diets.

Many people are confused about the concept and importance of calories. We **CANNOT** manipulate or outsmart the biology and physics associated with caloric intake, so think of calories as the **god of your fat loss efforts.** If you **FOLLOW ONLY ONE OF OUR RULES,** make it this one. Now, let's explore calories in layman's terms.

Firstly, you should know that your body needs energy to work. Just like a car needs gas to drive, your body needs fuel to keep your heart beating, your lungs functioning, your bladder working, and your brain going. It needs to use even more fuel if you're working out or playing sports. Every part of your body requires energy — without it, you would die. Even blinking takes up energy!

In a simplistic dieter's scenario, your body can get energy from two places: food (in the way of calories) or stored fat. Thus, if you don't give your body enough food for the day, it will tap into its stored fat to keep it going (the fat is burned up for energy). If you give it too much outside fuel (food), it will use what it needs and store the rest as pure fat, just in case it needs to pull from those fat reserves again in times you don't eat enough, or in times of starvation.

If you're reading this book, we doubt you have a serious problem with starvation, therefore you don't need all the extra fat hanging around for a time when you aren't catching any buffalo. We're not cavemen anymore, thankfully!

Remember, food is a source of fuel. Just like we said previously, your body doesn't care how good or bad food tastes. Whether you eat broccoli with a happy face or a disgusted face, your body will utilize the calories the exact same way. The only reason you eat junk food is for yourself and your own pleasure. The mind is what craves and wants junk food, not the body. We'll talk about the *type* of calories you should be eating later, but here is how you find the *amount* of calories you should be eating.

To find out how many calories you need to lose, maintain, or gain weight you have to know 3 things: your BMR, activity level, and your goals for your body. By knowing and calculating your daily caloric intake you will become much more aware and accountable with your consumption of food.

Your BMR (Basal Metabolic Rate) is the amount of calories you burn when at rest. So if you stayed in bed all day, your body would burn this amount of calories just to keep you alive. Things like aiding your digestive system, heart, lungs, brain, nervous system, and entire body to function properly uses calories. To find your BMR, use the Mifflin-St. Jeor equation. Break out that calculator and pen and paper, it's time to solve the equation for your new lifestyle!

This equation requires weight in **kilograms (pounds divided by 2.2),** height in **centimeters (inches multiplied by 2.54),** and your age in years.

Mifflin-St. Jeor Equation

Women: BMR = (10 x weight) + (6.25 x height) − (5 x age) − 161

Men: BMR = (10 x weight) + (6.25 x height) − (5 x age)

Once you find your BMR, you then have to calculate how many calories **YOU ACTUALLY** burn throughout the day since you aren't going to be spending your entire day in bed. Make sure you don't **OVERESTIMATE** your daily activity — be honest with yourself!

- **Sedentary** (little or no exercise) : BMR x 1.2

- **Lightly Active** (light exercise/sports 1-4 days a week) – BMR x 1.375

- **Moderately Active** (moderate exercise/sports 4-6 days a week) – BMR x 1.55

- **Very Active** (hard exercise/sports 6-7 days a week) – BMR x 1.725

- **Extra Active** (very hard exercise/sports AND physical job or 2x training) – BMR x 1.9

Now that you know how many calories you burn a day, let's look at your goals.

To Lose Weight: Eat 500 – 2,000 calories **LESS** than you burn a day. But, **NEVER** go less than 1,100 calories a day total for men and women.

To Gain Weight: Eat 250 - 1,200 calories **MORE** than you burn a day. You must also weight train very intensely and frequently if your goal is muscle gain (bodybuilding, sports, etc.)

To Maintain Weight: Eat equal amount of calories you burn.

*Note: 1lb of bodyweight is roughly 3,500 calories

EXAMPLE:

A 35yr old, lightly active (walks 3 days a week), 5'7", 240lb woman wants to lose weight.

o Her BMR (by using the formula above) is 1,819 calories.

o To calculate her total daily calorie expenditure with her lightly active lifestyle, she burns 2,183 calories a day.

o To lose weight, she will be adventurous and eat 1,083 calories a day **UNDER** the amount of daily calories she expends, which means she'll be eating 1,100 calories a day.

o This is a calorie deficit of 1,083 calories a day. For an entire 7-day week, this is a weekly deficit of 7,581 calories! As we said before, 3,500 calories equals a pound, which means she will lose over 2lbs of **PURE FAT** this week, even more if she exercises harder or more frequently!

o Because of her reduced caloric intake, healthier and cleaner eating, and following the Finale Lifestyle, she could lose over

5lbs a week for the first few weeks or months and steadily lose 2lbs a week until she wants to maintain her weight. This is not only based on calories, but based on the combination of a reduced caloric intake, healthier foods, and a more positive lifestyle. She'll lose more than just fat; she'll lose water, won't be as bloated, and her body will be more efficient!

Each meal should consist of at least 300 calories, and every snack should be at least 100 calories. To break them up equally, take your total caloric intake and subtract **AT LEAST** 200 calories for your two snacks of the day (100 calories each), divide the new number by 3, and that will be the calories for each meal.

For instance, if someone is eating 1,500 calories a day and their two snacks are 150 calories, they will have 400 calories for each of their 3 main meals. The lowest you should go is 1,100 calories a day, which is why we say every meal should be at least 300 calories and each snack should be 100 calories; that's a total of 1,100 calories a day. Always remember, Math = weight loss! Again, this is just an example to provide you with the process of figuring out this calorie rule. It's fairly simple and straightforward. Whether you are a male trying to gain muscle or lose fat, or a woman trying to maintain or lose weight, this formula will work. Remember, calories are important, so important you must keep track of everything that you eat.

This way you know how many calories you are putting into your body. Eventually, you may be able to be a little less specific because of your expanded knowledge on the foods you frequently eat, but for now make sure you are calculating everything correctly and perfectly so you achieve your goals!

Make sure you reassess your caloric intake every week. For example, every Sunday make sure your calories still match your current weight. The more weight you lose, the fewer calories you will need, and you must readjust. The opposite is also true.

2. Every Meal Rule

Every meal consists of Protein, Carbohydrate, and Fruit and/or Vegetable

EVERY MEAL should consist of a Protein, Carbohydrate, and Fruit and/or Vegetable. This ensures you have a great balance of macronutrients. Following this rule, we will show you what to look for in each protein and carbohydrate in your meal, and the exact portion sizes will be determined by your caloric intake and dietary preferences. Always remember your meals can contain more than 1 protein, carb, fruit, or veggie but should contain **at least 1** of each (protein, carb) and 1 or both of (fruit, veggie).

Also, it's important to note that dairy products like skim / low-fat milk can be used as the main source of protein. Things like low-fat / fat-free cheese are usually added to meals for flavor, and can serve as a "double protein" on a chicken breast, plate of spaghetti and sausage, chicken pizza, etc.

All of this is fine as long as you track the calories and everything fits within the 10 Rules for Life. Here, we give you a few examples of the types of meals you will be eating with Finale. We also substituted the protein for a dairy product on the first example of breakfast to show you how you could use them as the main source of protein if you're not a big meat person.

So, a great breakfast would be as such:

Protein: Skim Milk

Carbohydrate: Oatmeal

Fruit: Strawberries

It could also look like this:

Protein: Egg white and spinach omelet

Carbohydrate: 100% wheat toast

Veggie: Spinach (in the omelet)

Fruit: Apple (optional)

Drink: Coffee (black) or tea

That's it! It's that simple. We suggest you
eat about 4-5 times a day. Breakfast, Lunch,
Snack, Dinner, Snack. But remember, you should
eat how frequent you want to. If 3 meals a day
is better for you, then that's fine, they'll
just be a little larger!

**A lunch or dinner could look something like
this:**

Protein: Boneless chicken breast

Protein: Fat-free cheddar cheese (melted on
chicken)

Carbohydrate: 100% whole grain brown rice

Veggie: Homemade salsa (topped on chicken)

It could also look like this:

Grilled chicken pizza

Carbohydrate: 100% whole wheat pizza crust

Protein: Grilled chicken

Protein: Fat-free mozzarella cheese

Veggie: Toppings like tomatoes, spinach, asparagus, etc.

Another lunch or dinner idea:

Chicken cheesesteak

Protein: Grilled chicken

Protein: Fat-free provolone

Carbohydrate: 100% whole wheat long roll

Veggie: Side salad

One more, using cheese as the only protein:

Quesadilla with side salad

Protein: Low-fat / fat-free cheddar & pepper jack cheese

Carbohydrate: 100% whole wheat tortilla

Veggie: Side salad

You could even have mac and cheese:

Carbohydrate: 100% whole wheat macaroni

(with low-fat / fat-free cheese)

Protein: Chicken or turkey breast with

panko crumbs / cheese in macaroni

Veggie: Broccoli

To assure you get the right nutrients, the first thing you must do is make sure you get your 1-2 servings of fruits and/or vegetables in your meal. After that, make sure your protein is 3 - 8oz. Then, the rest of the available calories in your meal should make up your carbohydrates. If you're not a big meat person you could choose a portion of meat closer to 3oz to get more carbohydrates, or choose a portion closer to 8oz to make up more calories from protein. That's your choice, but we recommend consuming both equally, as both proteins and carbohydrates have immense health and fitness benefits.

We try to simplify Finale as much as we can so you can succeed! Could you ask for anything better!? You don't have to stick to a diet; you don't have to be confined with your options! Use this guide when you eat out and ask for nutritional facts to make sure the restaurants have protein and carbohydrate options that meet the rules of Finale!

Most of our followers tell us how amazing the flexibility is. So go to your favorite restaurant and order your favorite lean turkey burger on a whole wheat bun, order a salad on the side as your veggies, drink a diet soda, and thank us later!

3. Carbohydrate Rule

**Protein AND Dietary Fiber > Sugars AND
Saturated Fat < 1g in each serving**

Applies to any food with more carbohydrates than
proteins (exclude dairy & beans)

Many people think carbohydrates are the
enemy. But really, carbohydrates are
EXCELLENT. They provide energy to the body,
fiber for your gastrointestinal system, fight
many different cancers, and are full of
nutrients like B vitamins, magnesium, and
selenium. Carbohydrates help us burn fat, stay
full, and increase our satisfaction with
dieting.

Carbohydrates aren't created equal. Carbs
in the form of candy aren't good for you and
provide no nutritional value. Don't worry
about this because candy bars, cookies, and
cakes won't be satisfactory for our
carbohydrate rule. You must eat the type of

carbs that fall under the guidelines of this carbohydrate rule. **Also, make sure at least half of the carbohydrates you eat are 100% whole grain or 100% whole wheat.**

Look at the nutritional label on your selected carbohydrate. Whether you're eating rice, bread, crackers, pasta, or anything else, **the protein must be higher than the sugars AND the fiber must be higher than the sugars. Also, the saturated fat should be UNDER 1g.**

We must reiterate, carbohydrates **ARE NOT** the enemy. In fact, if you're working out a lot, carbohydrates are essential to your workouts and your energy levels. You must eat carbohydrates to be able to work out hard and perform the exercises that burn the most calories and help transform your body.

Nutrition Facts

Serving Size 1 (46g)

Amount Per Serving

Calories 100

% Daily Values*

Total Fat 2g	**3%**
Saturated Fat 0g	**0%**
Trans Fat 0g	
Sodium 80mg	**3%**
Total Carbohydrate 24g	**8%**
Dietary Fiber 5g	**20%**
Sugars 1g	
Protein 4g	**8%**

*Percent Daily Values are based on a 2,000 calorie diet.

This is the perfect example of a carbohydrate. It has much more fiber and protein than sugars. It also has 0g of saturated fat. This is an awesome choice. If the sugars were 10g, this wouldn't be a good choice. The sugar to protein/fiber ratio would be out of hand. Also, if it had 1g or more of saturated fat, it's most likely not a natural carbohydrate and has been flavored with fat and/or fried.

Great ideas for healthy carbohydrates include oatmeal, grits, 100% whole grain rice, bread, pasta, lentils, beans, potatoes, and sweet potatoes. There are many, many forms of other healthy carbohydrates and you are encouraged to try them — just make sure they fit the rule!

Again, carbohydrates are excellent and absolutely imperative for your success at looking and feeling your best. Anyone who tells you that you must stick to a low carb diet is absolutely wrong and promoting unsafe and unnecessary diet practices.

*Note – All carbohydrates should contain AT LEAST 2g of fiber and protein

4. Protein Rule

**Saturated Fat ≤ 3.5g in a 3 – 8 oz. serving
(NO PROCESSED MEAT)**

Applies to any food with more proteins than carbohydrates (includes dairy & beans)

Protein is the building block of every cell in the body. You could not build and repair bones, muscles, skin, and even blood without protein in your body. It's very important to get adequate protein because there is absolutely no place for your body to store extra protein. It can't call on protein when it randomly needs it, which means it's very, very essential to get protein from lean, healthy sources every day.

As you can probably tell, there is protein in carbohydrates! In fact, beans are a great source of protein and one of the leanest sources to get protein from. Whole wheat bread can sometimes be fortified with protein, and naturally has about 2-3g of it.

To meet your protein needs you have to ensure that you get a decent dose of it at every single meal. All of your meals should have a serving of a high protein food such as lean meat, fish, beans, or fat-free / low-fat dairy. Each serving of protein should be kept to 3 - 8oz and all of your protein products for meals should contain less than 3.5g of saturated fat in these serving sizes. To make sure you are eating 3 - 8oz, weigh your foods on a food scale while they are uncooked. If you don't have a food scale, make sure you check out the serving size on the nutrition information label and adjust how many servings you eat accordingly.

Most people like to cook their food in the beginning of the week to make life easier during the week. That's fine, the only obstacle is knowing how much meat you're actually consuming since uncooked and cooked meat can vary in weight significantly. Follow these guidelines to ensure you know **EXACTLY**

how much meat to consume if you're cooking it
in bulk.

1. Weigh and record the weight of the
   meat (uncooked)

2. Cook your meat

3. Put the meat back on the scale and
   weigh it cooked

4. Divide the cooked weight by the
   uncooked weight

5. Multiply the number you got from step
   4 with the amount of ounces of meat
   you actually want to consume

6. Now you have the amount of cooked meat
   you must eat to equal the amount of
   uncooked meat you need to consume. For
   instance, someone looking to eat 6oz
   of beef may end up eating 4.8oz of
   COOKED meat (since meats lose some
   weight through the cooking process)

Nutrition Facts

Serving Size 1 (115g)

Amount Per Serving

Calories 100

	% Daily Values*
Total Fat 2g	3%
Saturated Fat 1g	5%
Trans Fat 0g	
Cholesterol 20mg	7%
Sodium 150mg	6%
Total Carbohydrate 0g	0%
Dietary Fiber 0g	0%
Sugars 0g	
Protein 18g	36%

* Percent Daily Values are based on a 2,000 calorie diet.

This would be an excellent source of protein! The saturated fat is under 3.5g — in fact, it's only 1g for 115g of meat (or 4oz).

If you are a big meat eater, you could easily eat two servings of this meat, making it a total of 8oz for 200 calories and 2g of saturated fat.

Also, eating red meat is fine. We're sure you heard the reports of it being linked to colon cancer, coronary artery disease, diabetes, prostate cancer, etc. You don't have to worry about this unless you eat it in large amounts **EVERY DAY** and alongside an unhealthy diet and lifestyle (in which anything is unhealthy). An occasional lean 6oz sirloin, asparagus, and a baked potato isn't going to kill a devoted, consistent, healthy eater, positive thinker, and daily exerciser. With all of that said, red meat should still be kept to under 20oz a week, and the bulk of your meat consumption should be from white meat like fish and poultry.

But, processed meats **SHOULD BE CONSUMED IN MODERATION.** Meats like hot dogs, bacon, sausage, and lunch meat like salami and ham have very high amounts of nitrates, nitrites, and many other cancer-related additives. Try eating natural meats such as leftover roasted turkey or chicken, not a meat sold in a container that lasts a month in the refrigerator. These processed meats should be eaten in moderation and ideally (but not always realistically) not at all . . . **ever.**

A few great sources of protein include skinless chicken breast, eggs, egg whites, turkey, tuna, salmon, sardines, low-fat / fat-free milk and cheese, and occasional lean beef. There are many, many other lean proteins available and you are encouraged to explore them — just make sure they fit this rule!

*Note - Protein for your snacks should be less than 1.5g of saturated fat per serving. The saturated fat rule above is for meals.

5. Sodium Rule

Sodium = Don't go overboard (over 2500mg) but don't obsess about it.

Sodium. Everyone knows about it. Too much of it bloats you, contributes to high blood pressure, dehydrates your body, and fuels the fire for diseases of the heart and diabetes. Or does it?

Sodium itself isn't that bad, it's high sodium foods that are troubling. Sodium itself doesn't directly cause high blood pressure, but when you couple that with high-calorie meals, processed meats, desserts, and absolutely no exercise, we have a serious problem. Usually a diet high in sodium is high in junk, because most fresh foods don't have a lot of sodium.

Most studies conclude that sodium intake itself has almost no effect on blood pressure and heart disease. That's right! Contrary to belief, sodium isn't killing us. Sedentary lifestyles, outrageous desserts, burgers with mayo, ham, and bacon on them, over indulgence in alcohol, recreational drug use, severe stress, and pigging out on calorie-laden meals

three times a day is killing us - not the
sodium in your salsa on your skinless chicken
breast!

As with anything, moderation is key, so if
you're still worried about sodium, 1,300 -
2,000mg a day is a lower level you can shoot
for (especially for individuals at-risk for
high blood pressure). Just because we say
sodium isn't going to make you drop dead
doesn't mean you should go and start pounding
salt on everything. Too much of certain
vitamins will kill you, too much water at once
will kill you, so we don't recommend having
too much sodium either. Staying at a decent
sodium level won't be hard if you follow the
10 Rules of Finale, and always be conscious,
but not obsessed, with sodium intake.

6. Fruit and Vegetable Rule

Fruits = 2 servings AND Vegetables = 4 servings. But more is better!

The tried and true foods for maximum health are no secret; they're the fruits and vegetables. Fruits and vegetables have offered a wide array of benefits for humans going back hundreds of years. There are no other foods you can eat that are as effective for your health and well-being like fruits and vegetables.

Fruits and vegetables are full of vitamins, minerals, and antioxidants. They **LITERALLY** fight cancer, disease, inflammation, macular degeneration, protect the heart and brain, regulate hormones and imbalances, boost immunity, and rid harmful bacteria from your body. The best thing you can possibly do for yourself is to make sure that you get your daily servings of fruit and vegetables every single day.

Examples of great fruits to eat are apples, oranges, kiwi, strawberries, blueberries, pineapples, bananas, watermelon, and grapes.

Examples of great vegetables to eat are broccoli, kale, tomatoes, brussels sprouts, carrots, onions, bell peppers, corn, mushrooms, and eggplant.

Getting your 2 servings of fruit isn't hard. Make sure you eat a serving at breakfast and another serving for snack throughout the day. You could also eat them with your main meals; it doesn't matter, just get them in! Eating a cup of pineapples with breakfast and a medium-sized apple after lunch would give you the 2 servings of fruits you need!

To get in your 4 servings of vegetables you could

: eat 2 servings at lunch and 2 at dinner

: eat 2 servings at breakfast and 2 servings at dinner

These are just ideas. You could eat some carrots and cucumbers (which could be a midday or nighttime snack) and that would count towards your daily servings. A cup of cooked spinach at lunch and a cup of cooked carrots at dinner is already 4 servings!

For added health benefits, try and make each serving of fruits and vegetables a different color. For instance, eating 3 oranges throughout the day isn't as good as having an orange, an apple, and some grapes. The same goes with vegetables: try broccoli, carrots, and corn instead of broccoli every time you eat your vegetables. They don't have to be different types and colors all of the time, but this helps you get the benefits from each unique fruit and vegetable. Be as versatile as you want, have fun with it!

*Note: 1 serving size of fruit is one whole medium-sized fruit or half-cup of fruit. 1 serving size of vegetables is 1 cup of raw vegetables or half-cup of cooked vegetables.

REMEMBER: Frozen fruits and vegetables are just as, and sometimes more, nutritious than fresh fruits and vegetables. We encourage frozen fruits and vegetables for longer storage, more versatility, less cost, and easier use and preparation.

7. Good Fat Rule

Healthy fats: Cook with & consume them daily

Who said fat was bad!? Well, we did. But certain fats are actually good! The saturated fats you should limit and the trans fats you should have **ABSOLUTELY NONE OF.** But, the polyunsaturated, monounsaturated, and omega-3 fats that are found in many oils, nuts, and fatty fish are important for your overall health.

These fats help improve and control blood cholesterol and insulin levels. They also protect the heart from irregularities such as disease and irregular heartbeats. They help prevent strokes, heart attacks, and play vital roles in the development and maintenance of the brain. As a whole, they are excellent for your overall health.

We recommend you cook and/or flavor your dishes with small amounts of olive oil, canola oil, flaxseed oil, avocado oil, pumpkin seed oil, coconut oil, sunflower oil, safflower oil, palm oil, or corn oil.

These oils, although healthy, contain a good amount of calories. Be cautious of how much you are actually using towards your cooking and be sure to count them as extra calories towards your entire day of calorie allotment.

In addition to flavoring and cooking with these oils, the best way to get good fats is to consume them through regular food. Almonds, peanuts, peanut butter, cashews, sunflower seeds, avocados, wild-caught salmon and sardines, albacore tuna, trout, and mackerel are great foods to eat to get healthy fats in your body.

Cooking with these oils, eating a tablespoon of peanut butter with your apple, adding olive oil to your bread or salad, eating a few handfuls of nuts a few times a week, and having about 6 - 12oz of salmon, tuna, sardines, or other healthy fat a week will be **MORE THAN** sufficient enough for your healthy fat consumption.

8. Beverage Rule

Water > Tea > Milk > Coffee > 0 Calorie Sweetened Drinks > Alcohol

And the obvious winner goes to **WATER**! How'd you guess? Water is amazing for many, many reasons. Water helps you stay full and lose weight, keeps your metabolism high, fights infection, prevents constipation by helping stool pass through your intestines, improves lung function, and prevents joint irritation and inflammation. A human could go about 3 weeks without food but can only go about 3 days without water, and that's saying they're already hydrated properly! Water is crucial, it's the oil to your amazing machine . . . **YOUR BODY**!

Tea is **AMAZING** FOR YOU. Green, white, oolong, and black tea are great kinds to drink. All four of these teas have outstanding benefits. Each one helps fight and prevent cancer, reduces and stabilizes blood pressure, calms and soothes the body, fights stress and depression, and boosts your immune system. They help make your gums and teeth healthier, your eyes clearer, they fight allergies, and aid your body in healing. We recommend drinking 1-3 cups of tea a day for maximum benefits.

Milk has always been great for you. It has tons of calcium to build healthy bones and contains a good amount of protein to help build, repair, and maintain muscles. It's also filled with vitamin D, phosphorus, niacin, and vitamin B12 which are all essential for maintaining healthy red blood cells, bones, and metabolizing sugars and fatty acids. Milk is also an amazing post-workout drink. Try to drink 1-3 cups of fat-free a day!

Coffee is sometimes looked at as the "it's 2am and I'm on the backshift" drink. Or the "I didn't get enough sleep and I need it" go-to. But actually, there are a lot of other reasons to drink coffee. Coffee is a great source of cancer fighting, immune boosting, mood elevating, IQ lifting antioxidants and compounds.

The reason coffee gets a bad reputation is because people are quick to load it with sugar and fattening creamers. Although great for you, coffee is not a necessity and does not need to be consumed if you don't like it or just don't care for it. But, for those coffee lovers, plain coffee is good in our book so go ahead and drink your 1-4 cups a day!

0 calorie drinks aren't horrible but they aren't amazing. Some say artificial sweeteners can trick our bodies by thinking we are getting real sugar, which leads to more hunger, cravings, and increased appetite. But some people control themselves much better and this **infrequent** effect is of no significance. We do understand that sometimes you want something a little different like a diet soda or a 0 calorie juice. We recommend keeping it in moderation if these 0 calorie sweeteners cause you to get hungry or increase cravings. Contrary to some belief, there is no evidence that 0 calorie sweeteners and diet sodas directly cause weight gain. A diet soda **IS STILL** better than a regular soda loaded with sugar.

Always remember, the artificial sweeteners used in today's mainstream products **ARE SAFE.** Sorry conspiracy theorists, but our government isn't out to kill us or give us brain tumors. Artificial sweeteners used in the mainstream market are **COMPLETELY SAFE,** especially consuming them in the quantities humans consume them in.

Having a few drinks a day of 0 calorie juices and sodas is fine. Although diet soda isn't horrible, the 0 calorie juices are recommended over them. But always remember, you **CAN HAVE** a few cups of diet soda a day if you must. It is 0 calories, and if it's going to keep you sane, you're better off drinking some diet soda than indulging in cake and ice cream or a regular soda. In any case, drink these 0 calorie drinks in moderation, water is still your best option!

Alcohol can have some health benefits such as reduction of heart disease, strokes, and decreased gallstone occurrence. Though not necessary or recommended if you already don't drink or can refrain from drinking, women can have a maximum of one drink and men a maximum of two. Any more than this and the benefits are reversed! If you can refrain from alcohol completely, that's better than continuing or starting to drink.

*Note: One drink is 12 ounces of beer, 5 ounces of wine, and 1.5 ounces of an 80 proof spirit.

The most important drink is water! Remember, your urine should be clear or "see-through." Once you start expelling dark urine, you know you're already dehydrated! To combat this, always have a water bottle on hand and drink occasionally. Exactly how much water you should drink depends on what you eat and drink overall. Drink more if you are sweating, exercising, and/or in heat. But above all, keep the urine clear and the feeling of thirst at bay!

*Reminder – Drink fruit juices in moderation. They contain a lot of sugar and calories. If you are going to drink these, please limit them to 1-2 cups a day and ensure the label specifically states 100% (orange, apple, grape, etc.) juice and "no sugar added".

9. Condiments and Flavoring Rule

Sugars < 6g per serving AND Saturated FAT < 1g total AND calorie total < 60 calories

This is a very important rule. Why? Because not many people like their burgers, steaks, and chicken plain, nor do they enjoy salad without dressing. So, what's the rule?

First off, you have to remember that BBQ sauce, ketchup, salad dressings, and dips can have **ENORMOUS** amounts of calories. Some creamy salad dressings have more saturated fat in them in just 4 tablespoons than double-burger meals at dine-in restaurants.

The less sugar, salt, and saturated fat, the better the condiment, marinade, etc. is for you.

o Mustard is a great choice. Regular mustard barely has any calories and flavored mustards are still fairly low in calories.

o Ketchup has a lot of sugar and calories. Aim for light / low sugar versions. You can also flavor and top your food with black pepper, hot sauce, hummus, and pesto.

o Salsa is an outstanding, low calorie, heart healthy option to flavor chicken, fish, turkey, beef, and vegetables.

o **A HIDDEN GEM** for flavoring is fat-free gravy. Most fat-free beef, turkey, and sausage gravies have about 30 – 40 calories for an entire half-cup! Just think about the satisfaction of pouring that gravy on your meat, rice and broccoli.

o BBQ sauce can be full of sugars and fats, so we encourage light versions with low sugar. Pick one low in saturated fat and sugar (as close to 0 as possible).

o Salad dressings can be filled with saturated fat, especially the creamy ones. Also, many have enormous amounts of sodium. Opt for a vinaigrette dressing or olive oil. If you do not like vinaigrette, pick a fat-free dressing with little sugars and calories.

o Regular mayonnaise should be avoided. Try
  low-fat or fat-free mayo and you will make
  out great.

o Panko crumbs or something comparable is a
  great way to change the taste, feel, and
  texture of your meats.

o As far as marinades and seasonings, pick
  ones that taste the best. Always choose
  ones lower in sodium (250mg and under) but
  again, don't be so cautious that you miss
  out on great tasting foods! Any marinade,
  seasoning, or spice with little sodium and
  no calories is great! As far as commercial
  brands, we would recommend seasoning with
  Mrs. Dash or something comparable. The
  reason for this is the great flavor and NO
  sodium or calories (which means you can
  flavor generously).

o Always try low-fat, low-sugar, and low-sodium ways to flavor food. Use spray butter or zero calorie alternatives to butter. Always remember — the lower the fat, sugar, and sodium, the better it is for you.

Remember: This is the category that can throw you off track of your diet. If the marinade, seasoning, condiment, or dressing contains calories, you must know exactly how much you are eating. This is where individuals lose track and end up eating way too many calories for the day. Track your serving sizes and **make sure you don't eat over 60 calories in toppings, marinades, etc.** We prefer you use spices and herbs to flavor your foods — that way you don't add any unwanted calories. Seasonings like Mrs. Dash have no sodium or calories and can be added to proteins, vegetables, and fruits generously. But once again, we all need to stay sane and it's OK to add BBQ sauce, mayo, etc. to your foods as long as you follow the rule of less than 6g of sugar each serving and less than 1g of saturated fat total. For all toppings and flavorings, **stay under 60 calories total**!

10. Snack Rule

Ideal: 1-2 servings of Fruit or Vegetable and protein *or* Healthy carbohydrate and protein

OK: Anything that falls within the allotted calorie limit of your snack

It happens. Midday sleepiness, late-night study sessions, and pushed back dinner times are a big part of our busy lifestyles. When this occurs, the first thing you want is a snack. First, try and see if you are **ACTUALLY** hungry. It's important to rule that out first.

Drink a few cups of cold water and see if you still need your snack since we mistake hunger for thirst **A LOT**.

If you are still hungry, it's time to pick a healthy snack. Ideally, we want you to grab a serving or two of fruits or vegetables with some added protein. Grab an apple with peanut butter, an orange and a piece of low-fat cheese, strawberries in plain Greek yogurt, or some cucumbers and carrots with fat-free ranch. Adding protein like peanut butter, cottage cheese, or Greek yogurt adds some variety to plain fruits and vegetables.

If you **JUST AREN'T** feeling fruits and veggies, you can try 100% whole wheat crackers, toast, or plain popcorn. Remember, snacks have to be either a carbohydrate and/or protein if it's not a fruit or vegetable and protein. Whichever one it is, make sure the carb fits the carb rule, and the protein is **equal to or less than** 1.5G of saturated fat. A few great snack ideas are:

1. Fruit or Vegetable
2. Fruit with protein (apple and peanut butter)
3. Carbohydrate that fits carb rule (Popcorn)
4. Another fruit with protein (plain Greek yogurt and strawberries)
5. Carbohydrate and protein (crackers and fat-free cheese)
6. Vegetable and protein (celery and peanut butter)

* For one snack a day, one of your snacks can be based solely on calories. For instance, if your snack is 150 calories, don't worry about the content of the food, just eat what you'd like and stay within that calorie limit. It's

important you try to go for something fairly healthy.

Brands we love include Fiber One, Kashi, Arctic Zero, Skinny Cow, Nature Valley, Special K, Yoplait, Chobani, and Quaker Oats. These companies make great bars, ice cream treats, and snacks that can fit right into your snack's calorie limits. 100-calorie packs are also great; if your snack is 200 calories, you could have 2! This allows for maximum flexibility and sanity! It's OK if you don't want fruits and vegetables for snack all the time; you're human. Once a day, opt for one of these bars, ice cream treats, or even your favorite candy, and as long as you stay within your snack's calorie limit, it's not cheating!

Bonus Rule: Cheating Rule

Yes we know this is your favorite rule by far. Even the most disciplined, hard-working fitness models, athletes, and performers need to "let their hair down" and enjoy some guilty pleasures. As humans, we are natural pleasure seekers and Finale **RECOMMENDS** that you cheat on your diet once a week for one meal. This can be breakfast, lunch, dinner or snack. We have more information on cheating on your diet later on!

Bonus Rule: Common Sense

This is an important rule. Common sense is what drives us as humans to make decent decisions throughout life. You already have common sense to help you through your dieting efforts. By using your common sense, you can answer all of the following questions correctly.

What is a better snack, a candy bar or a banana?

What is a better lunch, stuffed crust pizza or a tuna sandwich?

What is a better breakfast, a donut or a bowl of oatmeal?

See, you **KNOW** what is healthy and what isn't. Don't make it harder than what it is. Remember, when you're following recipes or adding things to food, use your common sense. If you are eating plain yogurt, don't hesitate to put strawberries and blueberries in it for flavor and to count towards your daily fruit servings. Use your common sense and you'll notice eating healthy isn't as hard as it may seem.

Things like frozen meals, although not
ideal, can be used sparingly in a pinch.
Fresh, real food is always number one, but
frozen meals can be great for convenience.
Always remember to subject them to the same
rules of Finale as your regular meals!

You should also make sure you are eating
foods closest to their natural state. This
means an apple is better than an apple pie, a
banana instead of banana bread, and
strawberries instead of strawberry shortcake.

Also, don't ever eat too much of a
specific food group. Boneless chicken is a
great lean protein, but don't go on an all
chicken diet. Fruit is amazing, but don't eat
10 oranges a day. Moderation and variety is
very important for overall health and
wellness.

Bonus Rule: SLEEP

We shouldn't have to tell you the importance of sleep. Sleep is essential to our health, well-being, productivity, and success. We recommend **AT LEAST** 6 hours of sleep, preferably 8. Although these are what we recommend, some people need more or less sleep to function well. You will have to judge the right amount of sleep for you based on the way you feel during the day. Getting restful, sound sleep helps our bodies recover, rejuvenate, repair, and be the best they can possibly be!

Diet Myths

Starvation Mode Myth

"Eat too little calories or don't eat frequent enough and your body will go into starvation mode. This means you will start to lose muscle and/or your metabolism will come to a halt."

We've heard it too many times! The problem with this statement is it suggests that your metabolism is based mainly on external factors. In fact, your metabolism is largely based on internal factors. As mentioned before, the majority of calories you burn are from keeping you alive! Things such as brain, heart, liver, lung, digestive function, and cell production use energy!

If you were to fast for 2 days (which we don't recommend for numerous reasons) your

metabolism would not slow down **SIGNIFICANTLY.**
You still will be breathing, pumping blood
throughout your body, thinking, and living.
Therefore, your body **WILL HAVE** to burn
calories in order to accommodate these
functions.

In order to do get the calories for these
actions, your body will metabolize stored fat
in your body and use it for energy. Once your
body fat is **EXTEMELY LOW,** your body will turn
into "starvation mode" and start eating away
muscle for calories when it's being starved.
Virtually all people aren't even this low on
body fat, and aren't starving themselves to
begin with. Low calorie diets that are high in
fruits, vegetables, lean proteins, and healthy
carbohydrates don't put you in "starvation
mode." They help you lose weight!

We don't recommend going under 1,100 total calories for the day because that **CAN BE** detrimental (especially if working out intensely). Although your body is amazing, it is important to fuel it with outside nutrition for it to remain **functioning optimally.**

So put this myth to rest. Only in extreme cases (extremely low calories with extreme amounts of exercise) or (extremely low calories with dangerously low amounts of body fat) will your body ever **noticeably** slow metabolism and/or eat away your muscle. After all, if this was actually true, fitness models wouldn't be so lean and fashion models wouldn't be so thin!

Eating Late Myth

"Don't eat late, especially after 7 or 8pm. The closer you eat to bedtime, the more likely what you eat will be stored as fat."

We laugh when we hear this. The truth is, losing fat isn't an hour by hour process, it's a 24-hour process. All that matters is how many calories you have eaten in a 24-hour period, **NOT WHAT TIME YOU ATE THEM.**

If a woman were to eat a lot of food (5,000 calories) all day but stopped at 7pm, she would gain **EPIC** amounts of weight. If a different woman didn't eat much all day (500 calories) because she was insanely busy but got home at 9pm and had a big dinner (600 calories) she would **LOSE** a good amount of weight.

We don't suggest you do what lady number two did, either. It is best you space out your meals decently (doesn't have to be exact) just for consideration of things like your blood sugar, sanity, and digestion. But what is for certain, is it **DOES NOT MATTER** when your calories are eaten, as long as you don't go over your daily calorie limit. So put this myth to bed, follow our rules, and you will be on your way to lean!

Eat Frequent Myth

"You have to eat every 2 hours to keep your metabolism stoked or you won't lose weight, you'll go into starvation mode, and you won't burn fat."

This is sort of in line with the first myth. Truth is, if you ate every 2, 4, or 6 hours there would be **NO SIGNIFICANT DIFFERENCE** in your weight loss. Your body isn't going to panic if it goes a few hours without food, that's ridiculous!

Even huge bodybuilders do not technically have to eat every 2 hours but they choose to because of the amount of food they have to ingest (sometimes over 5,000 calories).

Again, we don't recommend waiting every 6 hours to eat. It's not the greatest for your blood sugar and sanity. Not to mention, you'll want to work out every day and will require some good nutrition throughout the day to make your workouts really count. But, this statement is a myth, a big myth at that!

Weight Loss Limit Myth

"Don't lose more than 1 or 2lbs a week. If you do, you're probably losing muscle and it's very dangerous to do this."

We'd like to laugh again. Losing weight is simple math — just look at the calorie rule! But that's not to say this:

When you eat cleaner, cut bad foods, and do better overall in your diet and lifestyle, you will notice an abundance of weight loss. Agreed, some of this is fat and some of this is water mixed with toxins that have been stored in your body from the horrible foods you have been eating. Eating and living better will also reduce cortisol levels (a stress hormone) that also keeps you bloated and fat. So although most of your weight loss will be fat, there will be a good amount of "guck" that you shake from following Finale.

There is no need to worry. You can lose any amount of weight your body wants to lose. Just make sure you follow all 10 rules and you will see **DRAMATIC** and **AMAZING** results.

Calorie is a Calorie Myth

"As long as you stay within your calorie limit, you can eat whatever you want, including junk foods."

This is technically true. If someone ate 2 candy bars (totaling about 800 calories) a day, they would lose large amounts of weight. But after a few days, if not 24-hours, your body would respond in negative ways. Your hormones, blood levels, heart, brain, and vital organs would start to go haywire with the lack of nutrition. You could start fainting often, not feeling well, and eventually die of malnutrition.

If you were to eat 800 calories worth of chicken breasts, eggs, oatmeal, broccoli, spinach, and fruit you would be fine. Again, this wouldn't be quite enough calories, but the point is you'd be **MUCH HEALTHIER** and in turn leaner by eating the more nutritious, whole foods.

800 calories of lean protein, fruits, and vegetables **IS NOT** the same thing as 800 calories of candy bars. **DO NOT EVER FORGET THAT.** Every calorie you take in counts. The person who eats 2,000 calories a day of lean protein, fruits, and vegetables and the person that eats 2,000 calories a day of candy bars, potato chips, and cookies will look **MUCH DIFFERENT.** Also, when you're eating less, you must remember that every calorie counts. If you're eating 1,300 calories a day, you must ensure you're giving your body the proper nutrition it needs to function optimally every time you eat.

Cleanse and Detox Myth

"I'm going on a cleanse or detox. It cleans out your body, rids toxins, makes you healthier, and makes you lose weight."

This one really makes us laugh! Firstly, going on a cleanse or detox is like saying you don't trust your body. Your body is **AN AMAZING CLEANSER AND DETOXIFIER** THAT NEEDS NO HELP FROM FAD SHAKES, DIETS, PILLS, OR POWDERS. Your liver, kidneys, digestive system, and immune system do a **WONDERFUL** job of ridding your body of harmful materials.

There is no way to replace the actions of your organs. They are there for a reason. The claims of cleanses and detoxes are generally untrue and very dangerous. **THERE IS NO NEED.**

All your body needs is great nutrition. That is all it asks for. It's built to last and help you for the long haul. **ALL YOU HAVE TO DO** is make sure you do your part and eat a great diet to provide it with the necessary nutrients to give it a boost. Do this and your body will last a very long time. The best way to detox is to let your body do its thing.

Gluten-Free Diet Myth

"Eat a gluten-free diet and you will lose weight, feel better, and be healthier!"

This myth is hysterical, and we refuse to spend too much time on it. The point is simple, **UNLESS YOU ARE GLUTEN SENSITIVE or HAVE CELIAC DISEASE, THERE IS NO BENEFIT OF NOT EATING GLUTEN.**

Products with gluten in them contain a lot of fiber, energy, and essential vitamins. **DO NOT** go gluten-free if you don't have a gluten sensitivity or disease; there is no reason to and it's only making your life more inconvenient and your food much, much more expensive.

Shake and Meal Replacement Myth

"Replace a few meals with a shake or meal replacement bar and lose (and maintain) weight loss."

Drink a few shakes a day and eat just one or two solid meals — sounds easy right? Not so fast. First off, we have teeth for a reason, to grind up whole, solid food. Also, think about the process of digestion. Without whole foods with **REAL** fiber, our blood sugar levels and digestive processes are not doing what they're naturally made to do.

Like every health expert reiterates, **WE NEED FIBER** for the health of our digestive system, which is why a high fiber diet protects against things like colon cancer.

Nothing, and we mean **NOTHING** beats a balanced, overall healthy diet. A meal replacement bar or shake can be OK on the go, but it still isn't the same as real food.

When it comes to vitamins, minerals, antioxidants, and other nutrients, nothing beats the bioavailability, health benefits, and digestion advantages of **WHOLE FOODS**. The vitamin A in a vitamin pill or meal replacement shake isn't the same as the vitamin A in a mango. Period.

Even if you did see success on a diet consisting of shakes and meal replacement bars, it's sort of false. Although it's great you lost weight, you now have to fight the realization that you can't drink shakes and replacement meals forever — it's not realistic.

The only true way to lose weight and keep it off forever is to learn how to eat solid, healthy, balanced meals and make good choices for your life and health. A shake, pill, or bar just won't cut it . . . ever!

Fad Diet Myth

A fad diet is any diet that promises unrealistic weight loss and/or a regimen that is not normal or traditional in real life nutrition. This means, any diet program that doesn't emphasize a balanced diet of whole foods and a reasonable caloric intake is a fad diet.

Never buy shakes, pills, or bars that claim they will help you lose weight. Whole foods, a balanced caloric intake, nutritious choices, and a more active lifestyle are **THE ONLY** ways you will be able to lose, and keep off weight.

When you hear words like detox, cleanse, meal replacement, or pills and shakes, put your **FAD DIET ALARM** on and run for the hills. Any program that suggests you buy food products other than whole, real foods is doing you a huge disservice.

A fad diet is also something that restricts a certain food group entirely, or to unrealistic and unnatural levels. Any diet telling you to drastically restrict protein, carbohydrates, or fat to basically 0g is a fad diet. You can't go your entire life restricting carbohydrates, protein, and fat to unnatural, abnormal levels! You have to learn how, why, and what to eat! That goes out to all of you **LOW CARB PEOPLE**! Carbohydrates help us burn fat, give us important nutrients, help us stay full, and provide us with energy. **DON'T AVOID CARBOHYDRATES**!

Ask anyone who is in their 90s or 100s and they'll tell you the reason they are living so long is because they live happily, and (for the most part) have eaten a balanced diet. No one in their 100s is going to say, "Oh, I'm 102 because I don't eat carbs," or "I'm 98 because all I drank was shakes, took diet pills, and went on cleanses and detoxes." When you look at it this way, you realize how silly fad diets are.

Slow Metabolism Myth

"I'm fat because I have a slow metabolism."

We had to save the best, and one of the most frequent myths, for last! The truth is, the heavier you are, the more calories you burn a day! Yes, that means the 300lb woman burns **MORE CALORIES** and can **EAT MORE AND STILL LOSE WEIGHT** than the skinny girl eating her pretzels and water.

The fact is simple, unless you have severe health problems or are experiencing complications and side effects from medicines or health procedures, the only reason you are overweight is because you haven't been exercising and watching your calories.

Here's a quick story about genes and slow metabolism:

A fit young man comes home from working out and he takes off his shirt to change. His overweight mother says "Wow I wish I looked like that, you have good genes." He looked at his mom and laughed. She said, "What?" and he replied, "Mom, we have the same genes, you gave them to me."

Ever since then, his mom has lost over 150lbs. She realized that she **was** fit before, she **was** at a healthy weight before, and she **was** at her best at one time. Life's events, stress, and depression literally packed pounds on her. The only reason she was overweight was because she allowed these things to let her neglect herself. And although understandable, it's something she finally changed! **FINALE.**

Secrets of Fitness Models and Celebrities

Fitness models, bodybuilders, and celebrities have some of the best bodies in the world. Though very impressive, they are all human. Ever wonder how your favorite celebrity loses/gains weight so dramatically between movie roles, or how the guy in the magazine got so ripped? Well, that can be you! These are everyday people!

Discipline & Pressure for Achievement

The biggest reason these people have such great bodies is their discipline. They are 100% committed to achieving their fitness goals. They will let nothing or no one stop them. It's truly a mindset (which we explained).

This discipline is sometimes motivated by the pressures public figures have in society.

If a celebrity is playing a superhero in his latest movie, or a woman is always on the cover of different magazines, their discipline can come from the pressures the general public puts them under to look a certain way.

Although these factors may be true, these people stay incredibly motivated. They treat their bodies like jobs. They take how they look and feel very seriously. Most of the general public do not. Remember, treat your fitness goals like your source of income: it's a must for happiness, longevity, and flexibility in life.

Low Carb Trick

These people aren't always honest. To look extra ripped and lean, a lot of fitness models or celebrities go on a low carb diet about 2 or 3 weeks **BEFORE THE GENERAL PUBLIC**

SEES THEM. When you go low carb, you lose a lot of water weight. This stops you from looking and feeling bloated, thins out your face and waist, and can get you looking a lot more muscular (if it's there) and lean.

Although this does work, it doesn't work for the long-term. Bodybuilders also do this before shows, and as soon as a show is over, they go eat an entire pizza and they are almost back to normal. You realistically can't keep up on a low carb diet. Too many great foods like fruit, oatmeal, and brown rice contain carbs and are essential to your health and well-being.

If you need to lose weight quickly and want to look a little better for a specific event, you can go low carbohydrate for about 2-3 weeks before. Count your carbohydrates and stay **UNDER** 75g of carbs a day. Make sure you monitor how you feel. A lot of people going low carb report feeling dizzy, lightheaded, weak, and tired.

Carbs are important, and although this low carb trick may work, it's certainly not a good idea. We suggest you follow our lifestyle so you can look good whenever you want, and don't have to crash diet just to look better for a few days.

Very Low Calories with Lots of Exercise

There have been reports of celebrities and fitness models eating dangerously low amounts of calories while working out at dangerously high amounts. Again, these are celebrities and fitness models and when they decide to embark on these dangerous routines, they at least have 24/7 medical supervision.

We **DO NOT** recommend doing these types of routines. They can be very dangerous to your body.

The Celebrity's Biggest Secret

The biggest secret by celebrities and fitness models is what we preach! Living a Finale Lifestyle enables you to be mentally and physically healthy and beautiful. Eating great foods, enjoying life, staying positive, and disciplining yourself with certain rules and guidelines are what makes these types of people so successful. Remember, these celebrities got to their great status in life and fitness because they consistently followed a set of principles to achieve their goals. We gave you 10 rules, now go follow them and be successful!

Cheating On a Diet

Cheating on a diet is a must. It allows for sanity, satiety, and honesty. Cheating on your diet will enable you to feel better about eating healthy. It will get your mind back to a place where you never thought it would be. You can cheat on your diet once a week and still achieve your goals with no limits!

Although you don't **have to** do anything special to cheat on your diet, we encourage you to follow one of these following cheating methods. These are amazing when you are on vacation and want to add a little extra cheat meal or snack. And if you're really serious, these are even great for when you're home and you take your "once a week" cheat meal. Utilizing these methods may virtually erase the damage done by the cheat meal.

Low Carb Method

Remember, carbohydrates are not the enemy. But, when you decide you want to eat that apple pie and ice cream tonight, you may want to "trade" or "bargain" some sugars, carbs, and calories.

If you are going to cheat on lunch, make sure you go LOW CARB (under 30g a meal) for the meals surrounding that cheat meal. So, if your cheat meal is a burger, fries, and a soda, and you're going to eat that for lunch, your breakfast and dinner could look like this:

Breakfast: 2-egg omelet with spinach, apple, tea

Dinner: Chicken breast, salsa, broccoli, water or diet soda

By doing this, it allows your
carbohydrate stores to level out. This makes
your cheat meal sort of "essential" to fill
your carbohydrate stores in your body. Think
of your carbohydrate stores like a glass of
water. By not pouring anything into it all
day, a little excess water won't make it
overflow. If you have been filling the cup
little by little all day, a little excess
water would surely make it overflow.

If you were to save your cheat meal for
dessert, you will eat a low carb dinner
beforehand, and a low carb breakfast the next
day. Again, this works wonders and basically
erases the effect of your cheat meal!

Low Calorie Method

The low calorie method is a tried and
true method. We all know that calories in vs.

calories out equals weight gain or weight loss. Although a calorie isn't a calorie, for one day you can use the small truth of this myth to your advantage.

We are sure that by now you know the calorie rule. If not, use the calorie rule to find out how many calories you need in a day to maintain your weight. For example, say you need to eat 2,000 calories a day to **MAINTAIN** your weight. Calculate the amount of calories your cheat meal will be. Say your cheat meal will be 800 calories. Subtract the amount of calories in your cheat meal from your maintenance calories (1,200 in this case) and divide them up before and after your cheat meal (all before if the cheat meal is the last meal of the day, like a dessert). So in this case, if your cheat meal was at lunch it would allot you 500 calories for breakfast, 400 calories for dinner, and 150 calories for both snacks. This doesn't have to be exact, just logical. This method allows you to enjoy your cheat meal but still get the proper amount of nutrition and calories from good, healthy foods. Following this method will allow you to stay in maintenance mode. Therefore you will not gain any weight whatsoever, and maybe lose weight (if you work out extra hard that day) all the while cheating on your diet.

Remember, if your cheat meal is for dessert, you would logically eat all of your good calories up until the point of dessert.

Everyday Cheat Meal – Vacation

This is for individuals on vacation. At Finale, we understand if you want to cheat every day on your vacation. **THIS IS LIFE**!

To do this, you will allot yourself a specific amount of calories all day whenever you'd like. First, use the calorie rule to find your maintenance calories. Say it is 1,800 calories: you will cheat with half of those calories (900).

To bring some health into the equation, make sure you still get at least 2 servings of fruits, 2 servings of vegetables, and some type of healthy lean meat for the day with the other half of your calories (eggs are good in the morning). This will allow your body to receive some good nutrition while on vacation, but still allow you to enjoy yourself. You **DO NOT** need to follow any eating pattern with your vacation calories. Just make sure you track them and give yourself a good amount to have fun with, and use the other half to eat some things that follow the Rules of Life.

The great thing about this is if you follow it exactly, you won't gain weight, and may lose weight if you work out a little harder than normal or your vacation is a physical, active one.

Everyday Cheat - Life

You can cheat on your diet every single day if it's small. To do this, you have to make sure you get all servings of your fruits and vegetables in. Then take 300 calories a day of "whatever you want" (donut, pie, etc.) and allot it into your daily caloric intake. If you have to eat 1,500 calories a day to lose weight, you will now use 300 calories for "whatever you want" and 1,200 calories to follow the rules of Finale. We don't suggest this method every single day, but it's a good rule to use if you are starting to slip off of your discipline, need a small mental break, or aren't ready to **FULLY FOLLOW** Finale.

A Controlled Cheat Day

Yes, you read that correctly. An **ENTIRE** cheat day. Remember we said all calories aren't created equal — they aren't. But as long as you don't eat more calories than you burn (whatever the type) you won't gain weight in the short term.

To have an entire cheat day, go to the calorie rule and find the amount of calories you need to maintain your weight, and then subtract that number by 200. Say you need 2,100 calories to maintain your current weight: you'll eat 1,900 calories of **WHATEVER** you want. That's right: anything you want! By eating 200 calories **UNDER** your maintenance, not only will you **NOT** gain weight from this cheat day, but you'll still be **LOSING WEIGHT**!

It's important to know that this should only be done once a week. But if you'd like, you could do it on the weekends (Saturday and Sunday) to give yourself more flexibility and allow yourself to eat out and enjoy your favorite foods. If you would like to embark on a cheat day to literally eat anything you want, go ahead, you deserve it!

We can't guarantee you won't feel like crap afterwards! Even on these days, we still suggest you work out and get some fruits and vegetables in. So there you go; just watch your calories and get back on track to fresh, healthy, whole foods on the weekday!

Cheating on a Diet (Regular)

If you choose not to follow these "damage control" methods of cheating on your diet, then just cheat on your diet! Only cheat once a week for one meal and get back to your healthy eating. If you cheat on breakfast, just go about your day like a regular Finale day. The same with lunch, snack, dinner, etc. Even when cheating, don't go overboard and make yourself sick. Eat a reasonable amount of a cheat meal and move on! Just remember, only stray away once a week and you'll be just fine!

The Psychological Cheat Meal

The psychological cheat meal is just that, all psychological and no damage done. To do this, you can eat "something fun" with a 0 calorie beverage. For instance, most popcorn falls under the acceptable carbohydrate rule. This means instead of fruit, your snack could consist of popcorn and a diet soda. Think about that! You can watch a movie tonight with the kids, with your partner, or by yourself and snack on popcorn and soda and not even count it as a cheat meal!

You could eat whole grain crackers and a 0 calorie sports drink — anything that falls under the Finale Rules. We have found frozen buffalo boneless wing products that have fit our protein rule. Just imagine heating some of those up with a diet soda! **You could also eat ANYTHING within 300 calories and a diet drink and it still won't count as your cheat meal as long as you only do THIS ONCE A WEEK.** We recommend fruits and vegetables for snack, but sometimes you just can't do it. If that's the case, have a **PSCYHOLOGICAL** cheat meal!

The Biggest Secret to Dieting

Let's face it. Controlling the amount and type of food you eat can be challenging. Dieting and losing weight can be time and energy consuming. After a few days or weeks, a diet may seem unsatisfying and boring. That's OK, the best way to deal with these natural feelings of a diet is to calorie cycle. Calorie cycling is the biggest secret to diet success!

Calorie Cycling

Calorie cycling is just what it sounds like: cycling the amount of calories you eat day by day, mainly to increase satisfaction. See, when you go on a low calorie diet you can become very, very bored.

Say for example you need to eat 2,400 calories a day to maintain your weight. You have decided to be adventurous and eat 1,400 calories a day to lose weight.

After a while, the 1,400 calories a day are going to seem mundane, not enough, and you may get tired of it. Hopefully not, but sometimes this feeling is just inevitable.

The best way to combat this is to increase your calories on **SOME** days, but still at a level for you to lose weight. So, instead of eating 1,400 calories **EVERY SINGLE DAY**, you could start eating 1,800 calories **twice a week**. This method satisfies your mind and body, tricks it into thinking it's getting a lot more food, and enables you to feel like you're treating yourself when really you're still losing weight!

This is honestly the best way to go about staying on your diet, especially at times when you are starting to feel like your options

with dieting and food selections have stalled.
We **GUARANTEE** the few days you eat 1,800 or
even 2,000 calories instead of 1,400 you will
LITERALLY FEEL like you're cheating — you may
even feel guilty! That's OK, don't, you're
just losing weight and calorie cycling, which
is one of the industry's **BIGGEST SECRETS TO
STAYING ON A DIET AND HEALTHY EATING PATTERN.**

Another great reason why calorie cycling
is valuable is because it allows you to keep
calories in the bank in case you bottom out.
If you're eating 1,400 calories a day and you
cycle that between 1,800 calories - when
you're feeling extra hungry, ready to give up,
and can't do it anymore on 1,400 calories, you
have a 400 calorie blanket you can use to
satisfy yourself with more food. This allows
you to keep your calories in check, your

mental state fresh, and your body at a state where it's still shedding fat.

Calorie cycling is a great technique to implement. The recharged and refreshed feeling is just what you need when you're in a battle against the bulge. It will also make your lower calorie days seem much more manageable. Go ahead and give calorie cycling a try, you'll thank us 50lbs later!

Diets are Beautiful

Let's take a quick break and acknowledge the amazing benefits a great diet has on your life.

By eating and thinking healthier, everything opens up in life. Things smell better, taste better, and look better. The world feels amazing. You feel and look amazing, your confidence is through the roof, your goals crystalize right in front of you, and the world becomes yours.

When your face gets leaner, your neckline shows, your stomach gets flatter, and your legs look amazing, you seem to have a different experience in life. Remember, you can do this. We believe in you. If we didn't, we wouldn't have you reading this. Keep it up!

Transitioning into a Healthy Lifestyle

Transitioning into a healthy lifestyle will certainly be different. **YOU** have to be different. You have to elevate your mindset, believe in yourself, and have faith in your ability as a strong willed human to take on this endeavor. Know that you are amazing; know that you can follow a few simple rules with your diet. Know that you can be the **BEST YOU** that you can possibly be.

If it all just seems too daunting, you can start with little things. Here is a list of examples:

1. Stop eating as much "junk" foods
2. Cut back or eliminate soda & sugary drinks
3. Start counting your calories to become more aware of what you're eating
4. Stop eating so many sweets

5. Start eating healthier foods whenever you can

6. Follow only a few Rules of Finale

These small changes will go a long way! Some people may need to do these types of small changes before jumping into the entire Finale Lifestyle. This is completely fine and acceptable.

You have to remember that transitioning into a healthy lifestyle, eating healthier foods, and limiting your calories is going to take commitment. If you're used to pounding donuts and sandwiches for breakfast, ordering pizza for lunch, having Chinese food for dinner, not thinking about what you're eating, and/or heading home to a few slices of pie, you're going to go through an adjustment period.

Whenever you cut calories, stop eating when you aren't completely full, or aren't consuming the same high calorie, fattening, sugary foods, you're going to go through some cravings and hunger pains.

A little hunger can be expected when refraining from your old lifestyle. When you are in a calorie deficit, meaning you're burning more than you're taking in, you **WILL** experience a small amount of hunger. You have to remember, **hunger IS NOT starving.** If you are eating 1,600 calories of lean proteins, fruits, vegetables, and healthy fats, you aren't starving! Your mind is just looking for something full of fat and/or sugar. After a balanced meal, being hungry is mostly psychological. Eventually, you'll get used to this feeling and it won't be hunger, it will be a feeling of health, lightness, and efficiency. Bombarding your body with bad food every few hours is a sure way to stay full, but fat and full of health problems. Remember, your mindset is everything. **You** can get through this!

Tracking Your Weight Loss

To track your weight loss, we recommend buying a scale and putting it in a very accessible place where you will see it every single day. By seeing the scale every day, you are constantly reminded about the goal at hand. How could you really eat that candy bar with the scale staring right at you in the living room?

Every Sunday morning, before you eat or do anything else in the day, weigh yourself naked (or with minimum clothing). If you do wear clothing, make sure you wear the same clothing consistently at each weigh-in to get the **EXACT** weight loss!

Only weigh yourself once a week in the same clothes (or lack thereof). Your weight fluctuates throughout the day and week so it's counterproductive technically and mentally to weigh yourself before your actual, consistent weigh-in.

Once you have your new weight, plan your meals, assess your calorie intake, smile about your great weight loss, and get ready for another killer week!

Exercise Recommendations

Of course you must exercise! Exercise is a vital component to the Finale Lifestyle. Exercise reduces and reverses stress, improves your brain function, builds self-esteem, improves cholesterol, fights diabetes, improves heart function, bolsters immune function, fights cancer and arthritis, boosts energy, helps you sleep, and keeps you looking great. This is just to name a few benefits!

Cardio Recommendations

Cardiovascular exercise is important. This refers to running, walking, jogging, jump rope, hiking, etc. Anything that keeps your heart rate up for a consistent period of time is considered cardio. To calculate your maximum heart rate, the formula is (220 - your age). Once you get that, try and keep your heart rate between 50% and 80% of that number the entire time. To check your heart rate, you can wear a heart rate monitor or check it manually by holding your hand on your chest or placing your pointer and middle fingers on the thumb-side of your wrist. Aim for **AT LEAST** 40 minutes of cardio a day, at a frequency of 4-6 days a week. 1 hour of daily cardio is the most ideal, and you can work up to that eventually.

On days when the gym seems boring and the weather is nice, head outside for a run, play tag with the kids, have a cardio session with your dog, or play sports with your friends. The gym isn't the only place for cardio; what matters most is you get some type of moderate-intensity cardio (at least 40 minutes / 4-6 days a week) for your heart!

Weight Training Recommendations

Weight training recommendations vary much more than cardio. With that said, **EVERYONE** should train with weights for at least 30 minutes, at a frequency of 3-5 days a week.

Now, if you are an aspiring bodybuilder or fitness model, this number jumps greatly. Bodybuilders may weight train 6 days a week at very, very high intensities.

Ever So Changing

Unlike diet, exercise isn't as much of a static issue. Exercise routines need to be altered, changed, and differed based on how you're feeling, performing, progressing, and responding to certain exercises. There are many different phases, factors, and types of exercises that could go into formulating a

program. For more tips on exercise programs,
the right ones for you, and great routines,
visit our website http://www.fitwithfinale.com
and go to the blog section.

A Day in the Life of a "Finalier"

Someone who believes in Finale believes in being as stress-free as possible. They try and look at the good in everything, the positive in the negative, and the opportunities in their failures.

Someone following Finale doesn't stress out about being a little hungry because they're cutting calories, doesn't think they'll fail, and doesn't get discouraged over minor setbacks.

A sample diet of someone following Finale would be:

Breakfast: Spinach omelet, 100% whole wheat toast, apple, tea

Lunch: Chicken breast with salsa, brown rice, and broccoli

Snack: Orange and 100% whole grain crackers

Dinner: 6oz sirloin steak, small baked potato, carrots, 2 cups of diet soda

Snack: Plain Greek yogurt with blueberries, a fun size snickers

On top of eating like this, they went to the gym and did 45 minutes of moderate cardio and 40 minutes of weights. They laughed, appreciated life, surrounded themselves with family and friends, and then laid down at night for a good night's rest. That's all it takes!

A Finale Overview

1. Every meal contains a protein, carbohydrate, and fruit and/or vegetable

2. Make sure each protein has under 3.5g of saturated fat for 3 - 8oz (under 1.5g for snacks)

3. Each carbohydrate should have more protein than sugars AND more fiber than sugars

4. Consume at least 2 servings of fruits and 4 servings of vegetables daily, but more is better!

5. Try to eat at least 8oz of fish (salmon, sardines, tuna) a week and cook with healthy fats listed in the "Good Fat Rule"

6. Never consume over 60 calories of condiments/flavoring in your meals

7. Use common sense when dieting. Try to eat as close to the rules as possible, but some foods are still "close enough" to meeting our carb and protein rules to be acceptable meals and snacks. Remember that one food, food group, or type of food won't instantly cure disease, nor give you one.

8. Consume processed meats in moderation. But don't be scared to enjoy a hotdog or two on a special occasion at the ballpark or cookout.

9. Cheat on your diet once a week

10. Exercise every day

11. Think positive

12. Live life, love yourself, and prosper

13. Follow our blog for daily updates and inspiration at http://www.fitwithfinale.com

Finale Meal Examples

Here are a few meal examples. You can certainly add any spices, herbs, or seasonings you'd like and use 0 calorie options like spray butter. The following ideas will allow you to focus more on a Finale Lifestyle, ensuring you get your protein, carbohydrate, and fruit/vegetable at every meal!

Breakfast

Meal 1 - Omelet

Protein: Egg white omelet (with spinach)

Carbohydrate: 100% wheat toast

Vegetable: Spinach in omelet

Meal 2 - Cereal

Protein: Skim milk

Carbohydrate: Cheerios (Add a Sweet'N Low packet and cinnamon for flavor)

Fruit: Apple

Meal 3 – Standard Egg Whites

Protein: Egg whites

Carbohydrate: Oatmeal

Fruit: Orange

Meal 4 – Pancakes & Waffles

Protein – Half-cup of egg whites

Carbohydrate – 2 frozen whole grain waffles/pancakes

Carbohydrate – ¼ cup of lite syrup

Fruit: Half of banana chopped up on waffles/pancakes

Meal 5 – Smoothie

Protein: Vanilla whey protein shake

Protein: Cup of milk

Carbohydrate: Banana

Fruit: Banana

ADD CINNAMON FOR TASTE

Meal 6 – Bagel

Protein: Low-fat cream cheese

Carbohydrate: Whole grain bagel

Fruit: Apple

Meal 7 – Egg sandwich

Protein: 1 egg

Protein: 2 pieces of Canadian ham (processed meat, eat in moderation)

Carbohydrate: 2 pieces of whole wheat bread

Fruit: Apple

Meal 8 - Breakfast burrito

Protein: Half-cup of egg whites

Protein: Half-cup of black beans

Protein: ¼ cup of cheddar cheese

Carbohydrate: 2 whole grain tortillas

Vegetable: Fresh salsa

Meal 9 - Turkey and egg sandwich

Protein: 1 egg

Protein: 2 slices of turkey breast

Protein: ¼ cup of fat-free cheese

Carbohydrate: Whole grain English muffin

Vegetable: Sliced tomatoes

Talk about getting creative. Be inspired by your favorite restaurants. Recreate popular items from big breakfast spots and use low-sugar, low-sodium, and low-calorie options and you'll notice your selections for breakfast are unlimited!

Lunch and Dinner

Meal 1 - Chicken breast sandwich

Protein: Chicken breast

Protein: ¼ fat-free cheddar cheese melted on the chicken breast

Carbohydrate: Whole wheat hamburger bun

Vegetable: Side salad of baby spinach

Flavoring: Low sugar BBQ sauce on chicken

Meal 2 - Italian Sausage

Protein: Italian turkey sausage (processed meat, consume in moderation)

Carbohydrate: Whole wheat hotdog bun

Carbohydrate: Baked chips

Vegetable: Side salad of baby spinach

Meal 3 - Turkey Burger

Protein: Turkey burger

Protein: ¼ cup fat-free cheese

Carbohydrate: Whole wheat hamburger bun

Carbohydrate: Baked potato wedges

Vegetable: Cup of mixed vegetables

Meal 4 - Steak

Protein: 5oz Steak (A1 or light BBQ sauce)

Carbohydrate: Baked potato (spray butter and light salt)

Vegetable: Asparagus cooked with garlic

Meal 5 - Tacos

Protein: Lean ground turkey (taco mix)

Protein: Fat-free cheese

Carbohydrate: Whole wheat taco shells

Vegetable: Tomatoes and lettuce

Meal 6 - Mexican chicken

Protein: Chicken breast

Protein: ¼ cup of cheddar cheese (on chicken)

Carbohydrate: Brown rice

Vegetable: ¼ cup of fresh salsa (on chicken)

Vegetable: Broccoli

Meal 7 - Spaghetti and meatballs

Protein - Lean turkey/beef meatballs

Protein: Low-fat grated parmesan cheese

Carbohydrate: Whole grain spaghetti noodles

Vegetable: Heart healthy spaghetti sauce

Meal 8 – Chicken Caesar salad

Protein: Sliced chicken breast

Protein: Low-fat grated parmesan cheese

Carbohydrate: Whole grain croutons

Vegetable: Bed of romaine lettuce

Flavoring: Low-fat / fat-free Caesar dressing

Meal 9 – Thanksgiving Feel

Protein: Chicken or turkey breast

Carbohydrate: Whole grain rice

Vegetable: Broccoli

Flavoring: Fat-free chicken/turkey gravy

Meal 10 – Salmon meal

Protein: Salmon

Carbohydrate: Sweet potato

Vegetable: Asparagus

The options are endless. Whether you want a tuna sandwich, tofu, or something different, it's OK! Just stay within the rules!

Snacks

1. Any fruit or vegetable

2. Popcorn and diet soda

3. Whole grain crackers and cheese

4. Apples and peanut butter

5. Celery and peanut butter

6. Orange and whole grain crackers

7. Low calorie / sugar protein bar

8. Cereal

9. Low sugar cookies

10. Anything that falls into your Snacks calorie limit

Putting it All Together

There you have it. Everything you need to succeed on your diet. You will never have to go on a fad diet ever again. That's over. No more struggling with your weight, this is it! We have formulated these rules and information so you can put it all together and achieve your goals. The end of this book is the start of your new life. Go live the Finale Lifestyle and be the person you've always wanted to become. **Thank you.**

www.ingramcontent.com/pod-product-compliance
Lightning Source LLC
Chambersburg PA
CBHW060500280326
41933CB00014B/2807